Heart Healthy Woman

A woman's Guide to Understanding, Conquering, and Thriving with heart Disease

Dr. Sandra Brooks

Copyright@ 2024

The content in this book is for general informational purposes only and is not meant to be medical advice. Its objective is to support and educate readers who are interested in learning more about heart diseases and how to manage them. It is advisable for readers to seek the advice of licensed medical professionals for personalized lung disease diagnosis, treatment, and management.

Table of Content

Chapter 1

Introduction

Cardiovascular disease is another name for heart disease. Any ailment that affects the cardiovascular system is referred to as heart disease. Heart illness comes in a variety of forms, each with a unique impact on the heart and blood arteries. But because of anatomical and hormonal variations, persons who are designated as female at birth are at particular risk. Women's heart health is a major problem, therefore it's important to spread the word about how heart disease affects them. Dispelling the myth that it mostly affects males; heart disease continues to be the #1 cause of death for women globally. In the United States and globally, cardiovascular disease (CVD) is the primary cause of death. 2019 saw 1 in 3 deaths worldwide due to CVD. That amounts to nearly 18 million CVD deaths in just that one year. In addition to chest discomfort, women are more prone to experience other heart attack symptoms and to experience heart failure symptoms because women's symptoms of heart disease can differ from men's, women might not know what to look for.

Types of Heart Diseases

Coronary Artery Disease

The most common type of heart disease is called coronary artery disease, or coronary heart disease. It starts when cholesterol and other substances build up in the arteries that supply blood to the heart, hardening and narrowing them. This reduces blood flow to the heart, depriving it of oxygen and nutrients, weakening the heart muscle over time and increasing the risk of heart failure and arrhythmias.

Atherosclerosis is the term for the accumulation of plaque in the arteries. Blockages in the arteries can cause plaque to burst, stopping blood flow and potentially precipitating a heart attack.

Congenital heart defects

A congenital heart defect is a condition that affects the heart from birth. Congenital cardiac defects come in a variety of forms, such as:

- **Atypical heart valves:** Blood may spill from valves or they may not open correctly.
- **Septal defects:** Either the upper chambers or the lower chambers of the heart have a hole in the wall.
- **Atresia:** There is an absent cardiac valve.

Significant anatomical defects, such as the lack of a ventricle or anomalous connections between the main arteries leaving the heart, can be associated with congenital heart disease.

Many congenital cardiac abnormalities only show signs during a routine medical examination and do not cause any evident symptoms at all.

Arrhythmia

An erratic heartbeat is called an arrhythmia. It happens when there is a malfunction in the electrical impulses that synchronize the heartbeat. The heart may beat abnormally, too rapidly, or too slowly as a result.

There are various types of arrhythmias, including:

- **Tachycardia:** In particular, a resting heart rate of more than 100 beats per minute is referred to as a quick heartbeat. Numerous variables, such as stress, high blood pressure, smoking, excessive alcohol consumption, using certain drugs, and illnesses like hyperthyroidism or heart disease, might contribute to this condition. If left untreated, it can result in consequences such as heart failure, stroke, or sudden cardiac arrest.

- **Bradycardia:** Generally speaking, this means that the heartbeat is slow—less than

60 beats per minute. Bradycardia may not always be a reason for alarm, but it might occasionally point to a medical condition. Bradycardia can be caused by an underactive thyroid gland, age, certain drugs, cardiac problems, and electrolyte abnormalities. Breathlessness, lightheadedness, fainting, exhaustion, and chest pain are some of the signs and symptoms of bradycardia.

- **Premature contractions:** These irregular heartbeats that happen before the normal heartbeat are also referred to as premature ventricular contractions (PVCs) or premature atrial contractions (PACs). PVCs and PACs are common and often benign, but occasionally they may indicate an underlying cardiac disease or other causes like stress, coffee, smoke, or some drugs.

Atrial fibrillation: The hallmark of this prevalent cardiac rhythm problem is an irregular, frequently fast heartbeat.

Someone may have a racing or fluttering sensation in their heart. Arrhythmias can occasionally pose a serious risk to life or result in serious consequences.

Dilated cardiomyopathy

The heart muscle stretches and thins in dilated cardiomyopathy, causing the heart chambers to dilate. In addition to toxins, arrhythmias, and previous heart attacks, genetics can also contribute to dilated cardiomyopathy. The heart weakens and is unable to pump blood effectively as a result. Heart failure, blood clots in the heart, and arrhythmia are possible outcomes.

The AHA states that it typically affects adults between the ages of 20 and 60.

Myocardial infarction

Myocardial infarction, another name for a heart attack, is the stoppage of blood flow to the heart. Part of the heart muscle may be harmed or destroyed as a result.

A coronary artery blood clot, plaque, or both are the most frequent causes of heart attacks. Additionally, it may happen if an artery suddenly contracts or spasms.

Chapter 2

Overview

The term "heart disease" describes a variety of disorders affecting the heart and blood arteries. Heart disease is the primary cause of death for people with AFAB, a fact that many people are unaware of. However, studies reveal that it kills silently. According to one study, even though they had numerous risk factors, only 50% of AFAB adults under the age of 55 who had a heart attack believed they were at risk before the attack. For this reason, it's critical to understand your risk and take steps to lower it. By giving women the knowledge and tools to empower themselves, this guide hopes to encourage early detection, efficient management, and a healthier lifestyle. It does this by giving women a thorough understanding of CVD, its causes, risk factors, symptoms, diagnosis, treatment options, prevention strategies, and advice for living with the condition.

According to the Centers for Disease Control and Prevention (CDC), the most common type of coronary heart disease, or coronary artery disease, affects around 6% of American women over the age of 20. As people age, their risk of heart disease rises.

Numerous disorders that might impact your heart and blood arteries are together referred to as heart disease. Among them are:

- coronary artery disease (heart-circumferential blood vessel blockages)
- Blockages in the blood vessels in the arms or legs are known as peripheral artery disease.
- an irregular heartbeat, or arrhythmia
- issues with the valves or muscles of your heart (valvular heart disease)
- congestive heart failure (issues with the heart muscle's ability to relax or pump blood)

- coronary vasospasm, or abrupt artery wall contractions
- issues with the tiny blood vessels that divide off from the coronary arteries is known as coronary microvascular disease.
- heart failure characterized by a lower ejection fraction (the heart's chambers not contracting correctly)

These disorders may arise gradually or as a result of structural heart defects present at birth (referred to as congenital heart disease).

How is the cardiovascular system different in women vs. men

Numerous sex-specific variations in the cardiovascular system have been discovered by researchers. Compared to those designated male at birth (AMAB), those who are AFAB may experience heart disease differently due to these intricate variations, which frequently occur at a microscopic level. Here are a few instances:

- **Anatomy:** Individuals who are AFAB have smaller heart chambers and blood arteries. They also have thinner ventricle walls, or pumping chambers.

- **Blood count:** red blood cells are lower in AFAB individuals. They are therefore unable to hold or absorb as much oxygen at once.

- **Cardiovascular adaptations**: A person's likelihood of experiencing changes in altitude or body position (such as abruptly standing up after lying down) is higher in AFAB. Sudden decreases in blood pressure may result from these modifications.

- **Hormones:** People AFAB tend to have higher levels of progesterone and estrogen, while people AMAB tend to have higher levels of testosterone. Your general and cardiac health can be affected by these hormones in a number of ways.

Chapter 3

Causes and Risk Factors

Age, sex, tobacco use, physical inactivity, obesity, unhealthy diet, excessive alcohol consumption, non-alcoholic fatty liver disease, genetic predisposition, family history of cardiovascular disease, elevated blood pressure (hypertension), elevated blood sugar (diabetes mellitus), elevated blood cholesterol (hyperlipidemia), undiagnosed celiac disease, psychosocial factors, low socioeconomic status, air pollution, and poor sleep quality are just a few of the risk factors for heart disease. Heart disease in women is mostly caused by a mix of genetic predisposition, lifestyle factors, and illnesses such as diabetes, high cholesterol, and hypertension. Preventing and treating heart disease at an early stage require an understanding of its causes and risk factors.

A number of significant cardiovascular risk factors, however, can be changed by medication treatment, social change, and lifestyle modification (for example, preventing hypertension, hyperlipidemia, and diabetes). Research has also revealed that certain sex-based differences in these risk factors, such as age, sex, or family history/genetic predisposition, are unchangeable. Additionally, there are some medical disorders that may increase your chance of heart disease. Among them are:

- diabetic hypertension, or elevated blood pressure
- having diabetes or high blood pressure while pregnant inflammatory conditions like lupus and rheumatoid arthritis premature menopause depression
- HIV-related preeclampsia
- autoimmune diseases
- calcifications in the breast arteries

Your risk of heart disease may be raised by certain lifestyle choices, including:

- being obese or overweight
- cigarette use
- prolonged stress absence of exercise

Additionally, having heart disease increases your risk of developing a variety of other illnesses and problems, such as:

- heart attack and stroke
- cardiac dysfunction
- heart attack aneurysm

Genetics

A person's risk of developing cardiovascular disease is increased thrice if their parents have the condition, and heredity plays a significant role in this risk factor. Polygenic factors or a single mutation (Mendelian) can lead to genetic cardiovascular disease. Even though these illnesses are uncommon, there are well over 40 cardiovascular diseases that have been linked to a DNA variation that causes the disease. Numerous heart conditions are classified as non-Mendelian.

Age

With the chance of having cardiovascular or heart problems roughly double with each decade of life, this is the most significant risk factor. 65 years of age and older are thought to account for 82% of deaths from coronary heart disease. The chance of having a stroke doubles every ten years beyond the age of fifty-five. The mechanical and structural characteristics of the vascular wall also alter with age, which results in decreased arterial compliance and arterial elasticity and can eventually cause coronary artery disease.

Sex

Compared to premenopausal women, men are more likely to develop heart disease. It has been stated that a woman's risk is equal to men after menopause; however, new evidence from the World Health Organization contradicts this, stating that "a female with diabetes has a higher risk of developing heart disease than a male with diabetes. "Compared to women with normal blood pressure who experienced no pregnancy difficulties, those with high blood pressure who experienced complications during their pregnancy have a threefold increased chance of developing cardiovascular disease.

Tobacco

Tobacco usage poses health risks not only from direct tobacco use but also from secondhand smoke exposure. Smoking is thought to be responsible for 10% of cardiovascular disease cases; however, those who give up by the age of thirty have nearly the same chance of dying as those who never smoke.

Physical inactivity

Currently, the fourth most important risk factor for death globally is inadequate physical activity, which is defined as less than five 30-minute bouts of moderate activity or less than three 20-minute bouts of vigorous activity each week. Adults with diabetes mellitus and ischemic heart disease who engage in 150 minutes a week (or similar) of moderate physical exercise can cut their risk of these conditions by nearly one third. Physical activity also improves blood pressure, lipid profiles, insulin sensitivity, blood glucose control, and weight loss. Its benefits for the cardiovascular system might be partially explained by these effects.

The percentage of persons aged 15 or older who were not physically active enough was 31.3% in 2008 (28.2% of men and 34.4% of women).

Diet

Cardiovascular risk is associated with high dietary intakes of trans fats, saturated fats, and salt and low intakes of fruits, vegetables, and fish; however, it is debatable whether or not these connections point to the same causes. Frequent eating of high-energy foods can raise the risk of cardiovascular disease and induce obesity. Examples of these foods include processed foods heavy in fat and sugar. Consumption of salt in food may also play a significant role in determining blood pressure and total cardiovascular risk.

The World Health Organization estimates that inadequate eating of fruits and vegetables is responsible for 1.7 million deaths globally. Evidence of a moderate caliber suggests that cutting back on saturated fat consumption for a minimum of two years lowers the risk of cardiovascular disease. Elevated consumption of trans fats negatively impacts blood lipid levels and circulating inflammatory indicators; hence, diets excluding trans fats have been frequently recommended. According to estimates from the World Health Organization, trans fats are responsible for over 500,000 deaths annually. Research indicates that consuming more sugar raises the chance of developing diabetes mellitus and is linked to higher blood pressure and unfavorable blood lipid levels.

Alcohol

Alcohol consumption at high levels is directly linked to cardiovascular disease. The amount of alcohol drank may have an impact on the complex link between alcohol intake and cardiovascular disease. A lower risk of cardiovascular disease may be linked to moderate drinking without binge drinking periods.

Cardiovascular risk assessment

The best indicator of a future cardiovascular event is pre-existing cardiovascular disease or a prior cardiovascular event, like a heart attack or stroke. In patients who are not known to have cardiovascular disease, blood pressure, blood lipids, diabetes, sex, smoking, age, and blood pressure are significant predictors of future cardiovascular illness. A person's future risk of cardiovascular disease can be estimated by combining these and occasionally additional measurements into composite risk scores.

When should I call a doctor?

In fact, the new primary prevention guidelines state that your chances of developing heart disease later in life are lower the earlier the risk factors for heart disease are addressed or prevented.

Therefore, schedule a meeting to talk about ways to avoid heart disease if you're worried about your chance of developing it. By utilizing the Healthline Find Care service, you can get in contact with a cardiologist in your neighborhood.

Many heart disease warning signals, such as weariness, dyspepsia, and dyspnea, are easily disregarded as common ailments or aspects of daily living. However, since a heart attack can occur unexpectedly, it's critical to pay attention to any possible warning indicators. It's crucial to talk to your doctor about any symptoms you may be experiencing, especially if you have risk factors. Heart disease can present itself in a variety of ways.

What are the risk factors for heart disease in women?

All people are affected by the traditional heart disease risk factors, such as high blood pressure (BP) and excessive cholesterol, regardless of the sex given at birth. In addition, several diagnosis and risk factors are specific to individuals with AFAB.

High cholesterol

Everyone is at risk for heart disease due to hyperlipidemia, or high cholesterol. People AFAB may be more at risk from low HDL cholesterol (the "good" cholesterol) than AMAB individuals 65 years of age and above.

Diabetes mellitus

Compared to people AMAB with diabetes, those AFAB with diabetes have a two–four times higher risk of developing cardiovascular disease.

High blood pressure (hypertension)

Over 60-year-olds AFAB are more likely than AMAB to have hypertension, but they are also less likely to have it under control. This is partially because of variations in:

- **Responses to treatment:** Adverse medication responses are more common in people with AFAB profiles. Finding and sticking to a good treatment plan may be more difficult as a result of these reactions.

- **Sodium sensitivity:** Your body becomes more susceptible to salt after menopause. In order to keep your blood pressure from rising, you must limit the amount of sodium in your diet even more than you already did.

Menopause

Your chance of developing cardiovascular disease is lowered by estrogen. But your estrogen levels decrease when you go through a natural menopause or have your ovaries surgically removed. As a result, your risk of blood clots, atherosclerosis, and excessive cholesterol is increased.

Obesity

When you go through menopause, you have an increased chance of becoming obese (body mass index, or BMI, greater than 30). Additionally, there's a greater chance of gaining belly fat, which studies have connected to an increased risk of heart disease. Two out of three AFAB individuals in the US are obese. Those who are AFAB are more likely to be obese than those who are AMAB (64% vs. 46% higher risk of coronary artery disease). For those who are AFAB, obesity almost triples their chance of having a heart attack.

Autoimmune diseases

About 80% of Americans with autoimmune disorders (including lupus and rheumatoid arthritis) are classified as AFAB. Every year, that number increases. A person's risk of heart attack, heart failure, and other cardiovascular issues is significantly increased by autoimmune illnesses.

Preeclampsia and pregnancy-associated hypertension

Preeclampsia significantly increases your lifetime risk of hypertension and/or diabetes. It also makes strokes more likely. A person diagnosed with preeclampsia has a 75% increased risk of dying from cardiovascular disease in the future.

Gestational diabetes

A diagnosis of gestational diabetes increases your lifetime risk of diabetes. Additionally, having gestational diabetes increases your lifetime risk of cardiovascular disease.

Peripartum (postpartum or pregnancy-associated) cardiomyopathy

Heart failure may result from the weakening of your heart caused by peripartum cardiomyopathy. Serious complications and even death may result from this illness.

Polycystic ovary syndrome (PCOS)

The risk of cardiovascular disease is increased by PCOS. Individual risk factors such diabetes, high blood pressure, high cholesterol, and sleep apnea are frequently developed by PCOS patients. Up to 5 million Americans who are of reproductive age may have PCOS, according to estimates.

Preventing heart disease in women

Generally speaking, identifying your risk factors and taking steps to modify them is the most crucial thing you can do. Your likelihood of developing heart disease increases with the number of risk factors you have.

You can lower your risk of heart disease even if you might not be able to totally prevent it.

- Regularly check your blood pressure. Work with your doctor to reduce it if it's high.
- Create a fitness regimen that suits your needs. Gradually increase your weekly moderate-intensity walking activity to 150 minutes.
- Get your blood sugar checked if you have any diabetes risk factors, such as obesity or a family history of the disease.
- Consume a diet rich in fruits, vegetables, lean meats, and whole grains to maintain good health.

- Avoid alcohol and items that contain tobacco.
- Check your cholesterol and, if necessary, take action to lower elevated cholesterol.
- Get help if you think you may have sleep apnea or if you actually do.
- Engage in regular exercise.

Chapter 4

Symptoms and Diagnosis

Women may not always suffer the same signs of heart disease as males. There are certain sex-based disparities in tests and treatments. It's critical to discuss your risks, symptoms, test results, and drug responses with your healthcare professional. Because of our distinct medical histories and societal contexts, there are situations where individual differences outweigh gender-based differences in significance.

The signs of a heart attack may be one of the reasons women pay less attention to them. Compared to men, women are more prone to suffer from non-traditional heart attack symptoms.

Among the most typical signs of a heart attack in women are:

- Instead of the more severe chest pain that men frequently experience, chest pain that feels like tightness or pressure may occur; however, in certain situations, there may be no chest pain at all.
- acute or unusual fatigue that may appear before other symptoms and give you the impression that you have the flu.
- pain in the throat and jaw, frequently absent from chest pain
- Upper abdominal pain or discomfort that may resemble heartburn or indigestion
- either one or both arms are experiencing pain, discomfort, or tingling.
- upper back ache with a possible pressure-like, burning, or tingling sensation
- feeling lightheaded or faint

As heart disease worsens, more symptoms of heart disease in women could appear. Depending on the exact type of heart disease you have, your symptoms may vary.

Later indications of heart disease in females may include the following:

- swelling in your legs, feet, or ankles
- weight gain
- problems sleeping
- your heart feeling like it's beating very fast (heart palpitations)
- coughing
- wheezing
- sweating
- lightheadedness
- indigestion
- heartburn
- anxiety
- fainting

Diagnosing heart disease in women

A doctor will initially inquire about your personal and family medical history in order to identify heart disease. Next, they will inquire about the nature of your symptoms, including their onset and intensity. They'll also inquire about your way of life, including whether you work out or smoke.

A doctor can determine your risk of heart disease with the use of blood testing. The most typical is a lipid profile, which counts triglycerides and cholesterol. In light of your medical history and symptoms, your doctor might order further blood tests, such as those to determine:

- degree of inflammation
- potassium and sodium concentrations
- numbers of blood cells
- renal function
- hepatic function
- thyroid activity
- some cholesterol markers and other specialist lipid testing

A continuous EKG or ambulatory arrhythmia monitor, which involves wearing a device that continuously records the electrical signals from your heart, may also be recommended by a doctor. You may wear this device for a few days or a few weeks, depending on your symptoms.

You might require more intrusive testing to identify heart problems if the results of these tests are unclear. Among them are:

- cardiac catheterization, which assesses the health of your heart.
- arteries implantable loop recorder, an arrhythmia monitor placed beneath the skin to identify arrhythmia causes (irregular heart beat).

Chapter 5

Heart disease treatment in women

A multifaceted strategy is needed to manage heart disease, including medication, angioplasty and stenting, or coronary bypass surgery, as well as lifestyle changes like eating a heart-healthy diet, exercising frequently, controlling stress, and giving up smoking. Women can collaborate with their healthcare professionals to create individualized plans for effectively managing their diseases by being aware of the various treatment options available to them.

Women can obtain the right care and therapy by identifying their symptoms and getting a diagnosis as soon as possible. Depending on the kind of heart disease you have, the course of treatment could involve:

Medication

Your doctor may prescribe one or more of the following medications, depending on the type of heart disease you have:

- Medication designed to lower cholesterol can help you have lower LDL, or "bad," cholesterol and higher HDL, or "good," cholesterol.
- Inhibitors of the angiotensin-converting enzyme (ACE) stop your body from producing angiotensin. A hormone called angiotensin has the ability to narrow blood vessels, which can lead to hypertension, or elevated blood pressure.
- ARBs, commonly known as angiotensin II receptor blockers, reduce blood pressure by obstructing the angiotensin receptor.
- Anticoagulants and antiplatelet medicines aid in preventing the formation of blood clots in your arterial walls.

- Aspirin is a blood thinner that, by preventing blood platelets from clotting, may help reduce the risk of a heart attack in certain individuals.
- A wide range of drugs known as "beta-blockers" function by preventing specific molecules from stimulating your heart.
- Calcium channel blockers work by preventing part of the calcium from entering your heart and arteries, which helps to treat high blood pressure.
- Nitrates function by causing your blood vessels to enlarge, facilitating easier blood flow.

In addition to medicine, heart disease treatment may involve the following:

- **Cardiac stent:** An inflatable coil of metal mesh, known as a cardiac stent, is placed into a constricted coronary artery to increase blood flow to the heart.

- **Percutaneous coronary intervention:** This surgical technique, formerly known as angioplasty, aids in opening the blood arteries that feed the heart with blood. Following an angioplasty, a heart stent is frequently implanted.

- **Coronary bypass surgery:** Coronary bypass surgery may be advised in more serious instances. Open cardiac surgery is required for this. A healthy blood vessel from your leg will be cut out by a surgeon and used to bypass an obstructed or damaged heart artery. A 2018 study found that women are less likely than men to undergo coronary bypass surgery.

Men and women handle heart disease differently, with some notable differences being:

- Compared to men, women are less likely to be prescribed statins and aspirin to prevent further heart attacks. Studies reveal that the advantages for both groups are comparable, nevertheless.

- Perhaps because women have smaller arteries with more small vessel disease or less obstructive disease than males, women are less likely than men to undergo coronary bypass surgery.

- Cardiac rehabilitation can help people recover from cardiac illness and maintain better health. But compared to males, women are less likely to receive a referral for cardiac rehabilitation.

Chapter 6

Prevention

Heart disease is the leading cause of death for women worldwide. You can lower your risk right now by acting. If known risk factors are avoided, up to 90% of cardiovascular disease cases may be averted. Women of all ages can learn how to safely use FDA-approved medications and devices to prevent and cure heart disease by using resources provided by the U.S. Food and Drug Administration.

To educate you on heart disease and other illnesses like diabetes and high blood pressure that might raise a woman's risk of heart disease, the FDA provides fact sheets, videos, and other web-based resources. Additionally, they provide the Heart Health for Women page, which links women to resources that promote leading heart-healthy lives.

"A lot of women are unaware that they have a higher risk of heart disease. Fighting heart disease in women requires an understanding that females may have certain risk factors and may exhibit unusual symptoms, according to Dr. Kaveeta Vasisht, associate commissioner for women's health at the FDA.

Everyone's risk of heart disease rises with age. Heart disease is more common in women after menopause, although it can also strike younger women. Every woman has the ability to make daily progress toward living a heart-healthier lifestyle. The best thing is that improving your heart health also reduces your chance of developing other illnesses like diabetes and cancer. Here are some pointers on lowering your risk and making wise health-related decisions. Modest adjustments can still be beneficial.

Don't smoke or use tobacco

Giving up tobacco use is one of the healthiest things you can do for your heart. Make sure to avoid secondhand smoke even if you don't smoke. Tobacco contains chemicals that can harm blood vessels and the heart. Because cigarette smoke reduces blood oxygen levels, blood pressure and heart rate are elevated. This is because it takes more effort on the part of the heart to pump enough oxygen to the body and brain.

Adopt heart-healthy lifestyle strategies

For a total of two hours and thirty minutes each week, doctors advise exercising for thirty to sixty minutes most days. Furthermore, since long-term stress can hasten the onset of cardiac issues, controlling your stress can help reduce your risk of developing heart disease.

Eat a heart-healthy diet

A nutritious diet can lessen the risk of type 2 diabetes, improve blood pressure and cholesterol, and protect the heart. A diet that is heart-healthy consists of:

- fruits and vegetables.
- legumes, such as beans.
- seafood and lean meats.
- dairy items with reduced or no fat.
- complete grains.
- fats that are healthy, like avocado and olive oil.

Reduce your intake of the following:

- salt or meals heavy in sodium.
- Sugar or drinks with added sweetness.
- extremely refined carbs.
- booze.
- food that has been highly processed, such processed meats.

- Red meat, full-fat dairy products, coconut oil, and palm oil all contain saturated fat.
- Trans fat, which is found in some fried fast food, chips and baked goods.

Maintain a healthy weight

Heart disease is more likely in those who are overweight, particularly in the middle of their bodies. Conditions that increase the risk of heart disease can be brought on by being overweight. Among these ailments include type 2 diabetes, elevated blood pressure, and elevated cholesterol.

The body mass index (BMI) determines an individual's overweight or obese status based on their height and weight. Overweight is defined as having a BMI of 25 or greater. It is generally associated with elevated blood pressure, cholesterol, and a higher risk of heart attack and stroke.

Your waist circumference might also be a helpful indicator of your level of abdominal fat. If the waist measurement is more than, there is an increased risk of heart disease.

- 40 inches (101.6 centimeters, or cm) for men.
- 35 inches (88.9 cm) for women.

A tiny weight decrease can still have health benefits. Even a small weight loss of 3% to 5% can help reduce blood triglycerides, a kind of fat. It has the ability to decrease glucose, or blood sugar. Moreover, it can lower the chance of type 2 diabetes. Reducing body weight further lowers blood pressure and cholesterol.

Get quality sleep

Individuals who don't get enough sleep are more likely to develop diabetes, depression, high blood pressure, obesity, and heart attacks. Establish a sleep schedule and follow it. Set your bedtime and wake-up timings for each day to achieve that. Maintain a calm and dark bedroom to facilitate better sleep.

The majority of adults require seven hours or more of sleep every night. Typically, children require more. Thus, be sure to obtain adequate sleep.

Get regular health screening tests

The heart and blood arteries can be harmed by excessive blood pressure and cholesterol. You can find out your numbers and whether you need to take action by getting screening tests on a regular basis.

- **Blood pressure:** Typically, routine blood pressure checks begin in childhood. Blood pressure should be checked at least every two years beginning at the age of 18. This examines blood pressure as a potential risk factor for stroke and heart disease.
- **Cholesterol levels:** Between the ages of nine and eleven, the National Heart, Lung,

and Blood Institute (NHLBI) advises beginning cholesterol tests. If you have other risk factors, such as a family history of early-onset heart disease, earlier testing can be advised. Screenings for cholesterol should be conducted again every five years following the initial test. Every one to two years, women ages 55 to 65 and men ages 45 to 65 should get screened, according to the NHLBI. A yearly cholesterol test is recommended for anyone over 65.

- **Type 2 diabetes screening:** Diabetes results in persistently elevated blood sugar levels. It increases the risk of developing heart disease. Being overweight and having a family history of the disease are risk factors for diabetes. Early screening may be advised by your healthcare team if you have any of the risk factors. Screening is advised beginning at age 45 if not. After that, every three years, you get your blood sugar levels checked once again.

Take steps to prevent infections

Cardiac infections can result from specific infections. For example, heart and blood vessel problems may be predisposed to by gum disease. Hence, brush and floss every day. As well, schedule routine dental exams.

Heart issues that already present can worsen due to other infections. Vaccines aid in the prevention of infectious diseases. Thus, be abreast of the following shots:

- Flu shot every year.
- The COVID-19 vaccine reduces the risk of severe illness.
- vaccination against pneumococcal disease, which lowers the risk of several bacterial infections.
- The Tdap vaccination offers protection against pertussis, diphtheria, and tetanus.

Ask your doctor or cardiologists if you need any other vaccines too.

10 facts you need to know about women and cardiovascular disease

1. Even though cardiovascular disease claims the lives of more women than all cancer types combined, just 44% of women believe that cardiovascular disease poses the biggest threat to their health.

2. Less than 50% of American women who become pregnant have good heart health, and approximately 45% of women aged 20 and over suffer from some kind of cardiovascular disease.

3. More than one-third of maternal deaths are caused by cardiovascular disease, which is the leading cause of mortality for new mothers. Maternal mortality rates are among the highest for Black mothers.

4. Preeclampsia, high blood pressure, and gestational diabetes during pregnancy significantly enhance a woman's chance for

having cardiovascular disease later in life. Overall, 10% to 20% of women will experience a health problem during pregnancy.

5. Although menopause does not cause cardiovascular disease, it does signal a time in midlife when women's cardiovascular risk factors can increase. For this reason, it is important to place more emphasis on health during this critical stage of life.

6. By education and lifestyle modifications such increasing physical activity, eating healthfully, and controlling blood pressure, the majority of cardiac and stroke occurrences can be avoided.

7. 51.9% of deaths from high blood pressure, also referred to as hypertension or the "silent killer," occur in women, and more Black women than any other racial or

ethnic group—57.6% of all women—have hypertension.

8. Even though there are currently an estimated 4.1 million female stroke survivors, women account for roughly 57.5% of all stroke deaths.

9. Because rescuers frequently worry about being accused of inappropriate touching, sexual assault, or harming the victim, women are frequently less likely to get bystander CPR.

10. Research and the STEM (science, technology, engineering, and math) professions continue to be underrepresented in women. In actuality, women hold 48% of all jobs in the United States, but only 27% of STEM-related jobs. Moreover, women make up only 38% of clinical cardiovascular study participants.

The End

www.ingramcontent.com/pod-product-compliance
Lightning Source LLC
Chambersburg PA
CBHW070440290526
45791CB00005B/2052